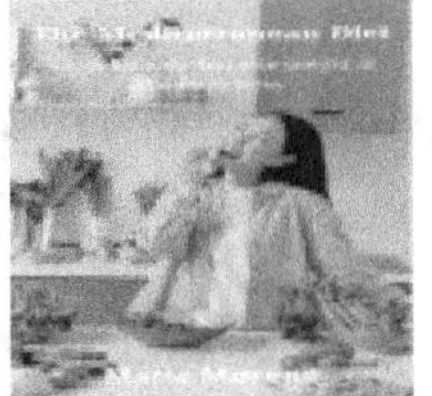

Introduction: What is the Mediterranean diet?

The Mediterranean diet is a way of eating that originated in the Mediterranean region and has spread worldwide in recent decades due to its numerous health benefits. The Mediterranean diet is based on a high intake of vegetables, fruit, whole grains, nuts, seeds and olive oil and a moderate intake of fish, poultry, eggs, dairy products and wine. It also includes a limited intake of red meat, processed foods and sugar. The Mediterranean diet has a long history and can be traced back to the traditional diet of countries around the Mediterranean, such as Spain, Italy, Greece and Turkey. These countries all have a common culinary tradition based on regional products and fresh ingredients. The Mediterranean diet is also strongly linked to the Mediterranean way of life, which has a cultural significance that goes far beyond nutrition. The Mediterranean diet has received a lot of attention from the scientific community in recent decades as it is associated with a number of health benefits. Studies have shown that the Mediterranean diet can reduce the risk of cardiovascular disease, stroke, diabetes and certain types of cancer. In addition, the Mediterranean diet has also been shown to protect the brain and reduce the risk of cognitive impairment and Alzheimer's disease. The Mediterranean diet is rich in healthy fats, such as olive oil and nuts, which help to lower cholesterol and improve cardiovascular health. The diet is also rich in fiber, which aids the digestive system and can help reduce the risk of colon cancer. The inclusion of fruit and vegetables in the Mediterranean diet provides a variety of vitamins, minerals and antioxidants that can boost the immune system and reduce the risk of infections. Another important component of the Mediterranean diet is the moderate consumption of alcohol, especially red wine. When consumed in moderation, red wine can have a positive impact on cardiovascular health and reduce the risk of heart disease. However, it is important to emphasize that excessive alcohol consumption is harmful to health and should be avoided. Overall, the Mediterranean diet offers a healthy and sustainable way of eating based on a variety of nutrient-rich foods. It is a way of eating that is based on pleasure and community and emphasizes the social importance of food.

The Mediterranean diet at a glance

The Mediterranean diet is a way of eating that originated in the countries around the Mediterranean. It is a plant-based diet rich in vegetables, fruits, nuts, seeds, legumes, whole grains and olive oil. At the same time, the consumption of red meat, sugar and processed foods is limited. This diet has long been the subject of research and has proven to be beneficial to health. The Mediterranean diet is associated with a reduction in cardiovascular disease, diabetes, obesity and cancer. Vegetables and fruit are important components of the Mediterranean diet. Most Mediterranean countries are fortunate to have a wide variety of fruits and vegetables that can grow due to their climate. A typical Mediterranean meal might consist of tomatoes, peppers, eggplant, zucchini, onions and garlic. Fruit is often eaten as a dessert or eaten as a snack between meals. Nuts and seeds are also an important component of the Mediterranean diet. They are rich in healthy fats, proteins, fiber, vitamins and minerals. Almonds, walnuts, pine nuts, sunflower seeds and pumpkin seeds are just a few examples of nuts and seeds used in the Mediterranean diet. Pulses are also an important part of the Mediterranean diet. They are an excellent source of vegetable protein, fiber and minerals. Legumes such as chickpeas, lentils, beans and peas can serve as a base for many Mediterranean dishes, including hummus, falafel and stews. The Mediterranean diet also includes a moderate amount of fish and seafood. These are rich in omega-3 fatty acids, which have anti-inflammatory properties and can help prevent cardiovascular disease. However, the Mediterranean diet does not include the consumption of meat and dairy products. Another important component of the Mediterranean diet is olive oil. It is used as a source of fat in many Mediterranean dishes. Olive oil contains monounsaturated fats, which are known as healthy fats and can help lower LDL cholesterol. In addition, the consumption of red meat is limited in the Mediterranean diet. Red meat contains saturated fat, which can increase the risk of cardiovascular disease.

Instead, plant proteins such as legumes and nuts are abundant in the Mediterranean diet.

The history of the Mediterranean diet

The Mediterranean diet is a way of eating based on the countries and regions that lie along the Mediterranean Sea. This diet consists mainly of plant-based foods such as fruit, vegetables, pulses and nuts, as well as olive oil and fish. The Mediterranean diet has gained popularity in recent decades, particularly because of its potential health benefits and its potential to prevent chronic diseases. The history of the Mediterranean diet dates back to ancient times, when people in the Mediterranean regions consumed foods rich in nutrients and fat. Olive oil was an important ingredient in many dishes, and fish and seafood were also an important part of the diet. The Mediterranean diet was more of a necessity than a choice at this time, as people in the regions around the Mediterranean did not have many resources to shape their diet in other ways. Over the centuries, the Mediterranean diet changed as people from other parts of the world visited the region and brought new ingredients and spices with them. For example, the Romans brought many spices and vegetables to the region and also introduced the cultivation of cereals and pulses. Over time, the Mediterranean diet became increasingly diverse. In the 20th century, the Mediterranean diet was first discovered as a potentially healthy way of eating. The discovery began in the 1940s when researchers noticed the low incidence of heart disease in Mediterranean countries. In the 1950s, Ancel Keys, an American scientist, launched one of the first major studies on the Mediterranean diet. He examined the dietary patterns of people in seven countries, including Italy, Greece and Spain. Keys found that people in these countries tended to have a longer life expectancy and less heart disease than people in other countries. In the 1960s, the Mediterranean diet was recommended by the World Health Organization as a possible dietary pattern. Over the years, further studies have been conducted showing that the Mediterranean diet is associated with many health benefits, including a reduction in the risk of heart disease, stroke, diabetes and some cancers. In the

1990s, the Mediterranean diet became increasingly popular with nutritionists and health organizations around the world. Numerous books and articles were published on how to incorporate the Mediterranean diet into your diet. There are now also many Mediterranean restaurants and cooking classes to help people try the Mediterranean diet.

The benefits of the Mediterranean diet

The Mediterranean diet is a diet traditionally followed by people in Mediterranean countries such as Greece, Italy, Spain and France. This diet is usually rich in vegetables, fruits, whole grains, olive oil and fish, and limits the consumption of red meat and dairy products. In recent years, several studies have shown that the Mediterranean diet has many health benefits. Here are some of the benefits of the Mediterranean diet: Reduces the risk of heart disease Heart disease is one of the leading causes of death worldwide. A large number of studies have shown that the Mediterranean diet can help reduce the risk of heart disease. One of the reasons for this is that the Mediterranean diet is rich in omega-3 fatty acids, which are found in fish and olive oil. Omega-3 fatty acids can help lower blood cholesterol levels and reduce inflammation in the body, both of which are risk factors for heart disease. Can contribute to weight loss The Mediterranean diet is rich in fiber and protein, which can help increase satiety and reduce cravings for unhealthy snacks. Some studies have shown that people who follow a Mediterranean diet tend to have a lower body weight than people who eat a different diet. Improves brain function The Mediterranean diet is rich in antioxidants and anti-inflammatory nutrients that can help improve brain function. A 2017 study found that people who follow a Mediterranean diet tend to have higher cognitive function than people who eat a different diet. Reduces the risk of diabetes Diabetes is one of the most common chronic diseases worldwide. A 2014 study found that the Mediterranean diet can help reduce the risk of diabetes. Another study from 2013 found that people who follow a Mediterranean diet tend to have lower blood sugar levels and a lower risk of diabetes than people who eat a different diet. May reduce the risk of cancer The Mediterranean diet is rich in fruits, vegetables, whole grains and olive oil, all of which are rich in antioxidants and anti-inflammatory nutrients. A 2017 study found that the Mediterranean diet can help reduce the risk of certain cancers such as breast cancer.

The Mediterranean diet compared to other diets

The Mediterranean diet is a way of eating based on the countries around the Mediterranean Sea. The Mediterranean diet has been the subject of research studies for many years to investigate its effects on health and well-being. Compared to other diets, the Mediterranean diet has many benefits and is one of the healthiest diets in the world due to its nutritional composition. One of the most important components of the Mediterranean diet is the consumption of fruits, vegetables, nuts, legumes and whole grains. These foods contain many vitamins, minerals, fiber and phytochemicals that play an important role in maintaining good health. Eating fruit and vegetables is also associated with a reduced risk of chronic diseases such as cancer and cardiovascular disease. Another important part of the Mediterranean diet is the consumption of fish and seafood. These foods are rich in omega-3 fatty acids, which have important anti-inflammatory properties and can reduce the risk of heart disease. In comparison, Western diets often contain too much meat, which is rich in saturated fatty acids that can increase the risk of heart disease. The Mediterranean diet also emphasizes the consumption of healthy fats such as olive oil, nuts and seeds. These fats are rich in monounsaturated and polyunsaturated fatty acids, which can protect the cardiovascular system and reduce inflammation. In comparison, Western diets often contain too many saturated fats, which can increase the risk of heart disease. Another benefit of the Mediterranean diet is the consumption of moderate amounts of red wine. Consuming alcohol in moderation can reduce the risk of heart disease, although too much alcohol can increase the risk of many other health problems. Compared to other diets, such as the typical Western diet, the Mediterranean diet has many benefits. Western diets often contain too many processed foods and refined carbohydrates such as white bread, pasta and sweets. These foods have a high glycemic index, which causes blood sugar levels to rise quickly and can contribute to a variety of health problems such as obesity, diabetes and heart disease. In comparison, the Mediterranean diet emphasizes the consumption of unprocessed foods and whole grains, which have a lower glycemic index and can help lower blood sugar levels.

What can I eat on the Mediterranean diet?

The Mediterranean diet is a way of eating based on the traditional diet of the countries around the Mediterranean and is known to offer numerous health benefits. This diet is based on the consumption of fresh and natural foods such as fruits, vegetables, whole grains, nuts, legumes, fish and olive oil. In this article, we will take a closer look at what should be included in the Mediterranean diet. The Mediterranean diet consists of a variety of foods that are rich in nutrients and antioxidants. The emphasis is on plant-based foods, especially fruit and vegetables, as these are rich in vitamins, minerals and fiber. It is recommended to eat at least five portions of fruit and vegetables a day to ensure a balanced diet. When it comes to fruit and vegetables, it is important to buy seasonal produce and use fresh, unprocessed produce wherever possible. Wholemeal products also play an important role in the Mediterranean diet. These include wholegrain bread, wholegrain pasta, wholegrain rice and other wholegrain products. Wholegrain products are rich in fiber, which plays an important role in digestion and can contribute to satiety. The consumption of wholegrain products is therefore an important part of the Mediterranean diet. Pulses such as beans, lentils, chickpeas and peas are also important components of the Mediterranean diet. They are rich in vegetable protein and fibre, which contribute to satiety and can stabilize blood sugar levels. Pulses can be used as a side dish to salads, soups or stews. Fish and seafood are another important part of the Mediterranean diet. Fish is rich in omega-3 fatty acids, which have an anti-inflammatory effect and can contribute to heart health. Fish is also a good source of protein. It is recommended to eat fish at least twice a week, especially fatty varieties such as salmon, tuna or mackerel. Seafood such as prawns, mussels and squid are also rich in protein and can be prepared as a side dish to salads or as a main course. Olive oil is the most important fat in the Mediterranean diet. It is rich in monounsaturated fatty acids, which can contribute to heart health. Olive oil is not only used for cooking, but also as a dressing for salads or as a dip for bread. It is recommended to consume around two tablespoons of olive oil a day.

The Mediterranean breakfast

The Mediterranean breakfast is a healthy and delicious way to start the day. It is a culinary tradition that originated in the Mediterranean countries and consists of a variety of healthy and nutritious foods. This breakfast is ideal for people who want to eat healthily, as it is rich in protein, fiber, vitamins and minerals. In this article, we will take a closer look at some of the ingredients and dishes of the Mediterranean breakfast. One of the most important characteristics of the Mediterranean breakfast is that it consists of fresh and seasonal ingredients. This means that there are different variations depending on the region and season. A typical ingredient is olive oil, which is rich in monounsaturated fatty acids and is used in many Mediterranean dishes. It is a healthy alternative to other oils and contains antioxidants that can reduce inflammation. Another important ingredient in the Mediterranean breakfast is bread. There are many different types of bread in Mediterranean cuisine, such as flatbread, ciabatta, focaccia and pita. These breads are made from wholemeal flour, which is rich in fiber and nutrients. There are also many other cereal products such as muesli, oatmeal and couscous, which are a healthy and filling addition to the Mediterranean breakfast. The Mediterranean breakfast also includes a variety of fruit and vegetables. Tomatoes, cucumbers, peppers and zucchini are some of the most popular vegetables that are often found in a Mediterranean breakfast. These vegetables are rich in fiber, vitamins and minerals and can be served as a side dish or in salads. Fresh fruit such as oranges, apples, bananas and grapes are also an important source of vitamins and minerals. The Mediterranean breakfast also includes a variety of dairy products. Greek yogurt is a particularly popular option as it is rich in protein and probiotic cultures. Cheese is also an important part of the Mediterranean breakfast and is often used in egg dishes such as omelettes or in sandwiches. Eggs are another important ingredient in the Mediterranean breakfast. They can be served in many different forms, such as poached, boiled or fried. Omelettes with vegetables and cheese are a delicious and filling choice for a Mediterranean breakfast. Drinks that are often served with a Mediterranean breakfast include coffee, of course, but also freshly squeezed orange juice, tea and water. Red wine is also an option, especially in Mediterranean countries, but should be enjoyed in moderation.

Snacks and small meals

Snacks and small meals are an important addition to our daily diet. They can help prevent hunger pangs and provide us with important nutrients when we are on the go or don't have time for a full meal. In this article, we'll take a closer look at snacks and small meals, examine their importance to our diet and recommend some nutritious options for daily use. Why are snacks and small meals important? Snacks and small meals are important to provide our body with the energy and nutrients it needs to function efficiently. If we go without food for long periods of time, our body can go into a state of starvation, which can lead to a slowing of the metabolism and a reduction in the body's ability to burn fat. Eating small meals and snacks can also help us to keep our blood sugar levels stable and avoid hunger pangs. In addition, snacks and small meals can help us to better control our calorie needs. If we eat smaller meals regularly, we can avoid overeating when we finally have time for a big meal. This can help us feel fuller for longer and help us consume fewer calories. What types of snacks and small meals are there? There are many types of snacks and small meals that we can enjoy. Some nutritious options are: Vegetable sticks with hummus or guacamole: Vegetable sticks are a great way to satisfy our craving for something crunchy while also taking in some important nutrients. Hummus or guacamole can help us meet our protein and fat needs. Fruit and nut bars: Fruit and nut bars are a great on-the-go option. They are easy to carry and provide us with a quick dose of energy and nutrients. Yogurt with fruit: Yogurt is a good source of protein and probiotics. If we combine it with fruit, we also get important vitamins and minerals. Quinoa salad: Quinoa is a good source of protein and fiber and makes a great base for a salad. Add vegetables, feta cheese and olives and you have a tasty and nutritious dish. Wholemeal bread with avocado: Wholemeal bread is a good source of fiber, while avocado provides us with important fats and vitamins. Together they are a great option for a quick meal. How can we make sure our snacks and small meals are nutritious?

The Mediterranean starter

The Mediterranean starter is one of the most famous and popular culinary traditions of the Mediterranean. This delicious and versatile starter is perfect for any menu and can be prepared in different ways depending on the culinary traditions of the region. The Mediterranean starter usually consists of a combination of fresh vegetables, herbs, cheese, olive oil and spices. Most Mediterranean starters are raw or lightly cooked and served cold. The best-known Mediterranean starters include caprese salad, hummus, tabouleh and antipasti. Caprese salad is a popular starter from Italy consisting of tomatoes, mozzarella cheese and basil. The tomatoes are cut into slices and arranged on a plate. Thin slices of mozzarella cheese are then placed on top. Finally, everything is sprinkled with fresh basil and drizzled with olive oil. Caprese salad is a simple but delicious Mediterranean starter that you can easily make at home. Humus is another popular Mediterranean starter made from chickpeas, tahini (sesame paste), garlic and olive oil. The chickpeas are pureed with the other ingredients in a blender until a smooth paste is formed. Hummus can be served on bread, vegetables or pita bread. Hummus is rich in protein and fiber and is a great way to enjoy a healthy and nutritious appetizer. Tabouleh is another popular starter from the Mediterranean region, consisting of parsley, tomatoes, onions and bulgur (cooked wheat). The ingredients are finely chopped and then mixed with lemon juice, olive oil and spices. Tabouleh is a refreshing and healthy starter that is rich in vitamins and nutrients. Antipasti is an Italian starter consisting of a combination of various Mediterranean ingredients. These include olives, sun-dried tomatoes, grilled vegetables, cheese and cold meats. Antipasti is a rich and versatile starter that is perfect for a buffet or party. Another popular Mediterranean starter is bruschetta. Bruschetta consists of toasted bread rubbed with garlic and topped with fresh tomatoes, basil and olive oil. Bruschetta is a simple and delicious starter that is easy to make at home. Olives and pickled vegetables are also a popular Mediterranean starter. Olives can be bought in many different flavors and sizes.

Soups and stews

Mediterranean soups and stews are an important part of traditional Mediterranean cuisine. With their versatility and ease of preparation, they are not only delicious, but also nutritious and healthy. Mediterranean cuisine is often referred to as one of the healthiest cuisines in the world, as it is rich in fresh ingredients such as vegetables, herbs and olive oil. One of the best-known Mediterranean soups is minestrone. The classic Italian vegetable soup is a delicious combination of seasonal vegetables such as tomatoes, zucchinis, carrots, beans and potatoes. The soup is often served with pasta or rice and sprinkled with Parmesan cheese. Minestrone is a great way to enjoy lots of healthy vegetables in a single meal. Another popular Mediterranean soup is gazpacho, a cold soup from Andalusia, Spain. Gazpacho is made from fresh tomatoes, cucumbers, peppers and onions and mixed with bread, olive oil and vinegar. It is usually served cold and is perfect for hot summer days. Fish soup is another classic of Mediterranean cuisine. Bouillabaisse from Provence, France, is an aromatic fish soup usually made with different types of fish such as sea bass, redfish, sole and octopus. The soup is seasoned with garlic, tomatoes, fennel, onions and herbs and served with a rouille sauce and bread. Another delicious fish soup is cacciucco from Tuscany, Italy. Cacciucco is made from a variety of seafood such as prawns, mussels, squid and octopus and is seasoned with garlic, tomatoes and wine. It is usually served with a slice of toasted bread. Another Mediterranean soup that is very popular in Greek cuisine is avgolemono soup. The soup is made from chicken stock, eggs and lemon juice and served with rice or pasta. Avgolemono soup is not only delicious, but also rich in protein and vitamins. In addition to soups, stews are also an important part of Mediterranean cuisine. Stews are easy to prepare and can be made from a variety of ingredients, depending on the season and the availability of fresh vegetables and meat. A popular Mediterranean stew is ratatouille from the south of France. The stew consists of eggplants, zucchinis, tomatoes, peppers and onions and is usually seasoned with garlic, olive oil and herbs such as thyme and rosemary. Ratatouille is often served as a side dish.

Mediterranean salads

Mediterranean salads are very popular in the kitchen and offer a variety of fresh ingredients and flavors that are easy to combine. Mediterranean cuisine is characterized by the use of fresh vegetables, herbs, olive oil and feta cheese. In this article, I will describe some of the most popular Mediterranean salads that are easy to make and perfect as a side dish or as a light lunch. One of the most famous Mediterranean salads is the Greek salad. This salad is made with tomatoes, cucumber, green peppers, onions, feta cheese and olives. The ingredients are cut into cubes and drizzled with a simple vinaigrette of olive oil, lemon juice and oregano. The Greek salad is not only delicious, but also very nutritious and full of vitamins and antioxidants. Another popular Mediterranean salad is the Italian Caprese salad. This salad is made with fresh tomatoes, mozzarella cheese and fresh basil. The ingredients are cut into slices and arranged on a plate. The salad is then drizzled with olive oil and balsamic vinegar and seasoned with salt and pepper. The Italian Caprese salad is a simple but delicious salad that is perfect as a starter or side dish to a main meal. The Turkish millet salad is another delicious Mediterranean salad. This salad is made with millet, tomatoes, cucumber, peppers and fresh herbs such as parsley, mint and coriander. The salad is drizzled with a simple vinaigrette made from olive oil, lemon juice and garlic. The Turkish millet salad is full of healthy ingredients and perfect for a vegetarian or vegan diet. The Tunisian salad is another

Mediterranean salad made with roasted peppers, tomatoes, onions, olives and capers. The salad is drizzled with a spicy harissa vinaigrette made from harissa paste, olive oil and lemon juice. The Tunisian salad is a delicious salad with a unique combination of flavors and spices. The Spanish Tomato Salad is a simple but delicious Mediterranean salad made with tomatoes, onions and olive oil. The tomatoes are sliced and arranged on a plate. The salad is then drizzled with olive oil and salt. The Spanish tomato salad is a perfect accompaniment to grilled meat or fish and is also suitable as a light lunch.

Pasta dishes

Mediterranean cuisine is known for its versatile and delicious pasta dishes. From Italy to Greece and Spain, there is a wide range of recipes that bring the taste of the sun and sea to the table. Here are some examples of Mediterranean pasta dishes you should definitely try: Spaghetti with seafood: This classic Italian dish is a delicious combination of seafood, tomatoes, garlic and olive oil. The spaghetti is cooked al dente and then tossed with a sauce of tomatoes, onions, garlic, chili and white wine. Garnished with mussels, prawns and squid and sprinkled with parsley, it is a delicious dish that is best enjoyed with a glass of wine. Fettuccine Alfredo: This dish originates from Rome and is one of the most famous Italian pasta dishes. The fettuccine is served in a creamy sauce made from butter, cream and Parmesan cheese. Simple and delicious! Spaghetti carbonara: Another well-known Italian pasta dish is spaghetti carbonara. It consists of spaghetti, eggs, bacon, pecorino cheese and black pepper. The eggs are beaten into a creamy sauce, which is then poured over the hot pasta. A simple yet delicious dish! Linguine with clams: This dish originates from Naples and is another classic pasta dish from Italy. The linguine is served with clams in a garlic and white wine sauce. The clams are cooked in a pan with garlic, olive oil, white wine and tomatoes until they open. The sauce is then mixed with the pasta and served sprinkled with parsley. Spanish paella: Although paella is usually served as a rice dish, there is also a pasta version. Fideos are thin noodles that look similar to spaghetti. They are cooked in a pan with seafood, chicken and vegetables and seasoned with saffron. A delicious and nutritious dish that is typical of Spanish cuisine. Greek pastitsio: This pasta dish is a Greek version of Italian lasagna. It consists of pasta, minced meat, tomatoes, cinnamon and nutmeg and is covered with a creamy sauce made from eggs and milk. It is a hearty dish that is often served at celebrations. Italian lasagna: This dish is one of the most famous Italian pasta dishes. Lasagna consists of layered pasta, minced meat, tomatoes and cheese and is baked in the oven. It is a rich and filling dish.

Rice dishes

Mediterranean cuisine is known for its light, healthy and delicious dishes. Mediterranean rice dishes are among the most popular dishes in the region and are often quick and easy to prepare. Here are some ideas for Mediterranean rice dishes that you can try at home. Paella is a traditional Spanish rice dish that is often prepared with seafood, chicken or rabbit. The rice is seasoned with vegetables, tomatoes, garlic, paprika and saffron and cooked with stock. The rice is then topped with the ingredients of choice and garnished with peas, olives and lemon slices. Risotto Risotto is an Italian dish made from Arborio rice, prepared with vegetables, Parmesan cheese and butter. It is creamy and tender and can be prepared in different variations. For example, you can prepare risotto with mushrooms, spinach, zucchinis or tomatoes. It is a quick and easy dish that always tastes good. Pilaf is a simple and delicious rice dish that is popular throughout the Mediterranean region. The rice is cooked in a broth made from vegetables, meat or fish and seasoned with spices such as turmeric, cinnamon and cumin. Pilaf can be served with chicken, lamb or fish and is often garnished with raisins, almonds or pistachios. Arroz con pollo is a Latin American dish made from rice and chicken. The rice is seasoned with tomatoes, onions, garlic and peppers and cooked with chicken and peas. The dish is often garnished with olives and lemon slices and served with a spicy sauce. Tabbouleh Tabbouleh is a Lebanese salad made from bulgur and parsley. The bulgur is mixed with tomatoes, cucumber, onions and mint and seasoned with lemon juice and olive oil. Tabbouleh is a refreshing and healthy salad that goes well with grilled meat or fish. Kuskus Kuskus is a North African dish made from semolina that is often served with vegetables and meat or fish. The kuskus is steamed and seasoned with tomatoes, onions and peppers. The dish is often served with lamb or chicken and seasoned with harissa or other spices. Dolma are stuffed vegetables that are often filled with rice and spices. The vegetables can be peppers, zucchinis or tomatoes. The filling consists of rice, tomatoes, onions, parsley and mint and is seasoned with lemon juice and olive oil.

Mediterranean fish dishes

Mediterranean cuisine is known for its fresh, simple and healthy ingredients. One of the main components of Mediterranean cuisine is fish. Fish dishes are very popular in many Mediterranean countries and there are countless variations to try. In this article, we will present some of the best Mediterranean fish dishes. Grilled octopus Grilled octopus is a typical dish in Greece, Spain and Italy. The octopus is cooked on a charcoal grill and then served with olive oil, lemon juice and spices. The octopus should be tender and juicy and the octopus arms must be cut into thin slices. Bouillabaisse Bouillabaisse is a French fish soup that is very popular in Provence. It consists of various types of fish, such as redfish, monkfish or Peter fish, as well as tomatoes, fennel, onions and garlic. The dish is served in a large pan with a rouille, a garlic mayonnaise, and a slice of bread. Calamari are fried squid and are often served as a starter or main course. The squid are rolled in flour, eggs and breadcrumbs and then fried in olive oil. They are served with lemon juice and parsley. Paella Paella is a Spanish dish that is often prepared with seafood such as mussels, prawns and squid. It is cooked in a special flat pan, a paellera, and seasoned with rice, tomatoes, onions, peppers and saffron. The dish is often served as a main course or as a starter. Cacciucco is a Tuscan fish soup made from various types of fish, such as redfish, monkfish or sardines. It is seasoned with tomatoes, onions, garlic and chili and served with a slice of bread. Fish in a salt crust Fish in a salt crust is a simple and healthy dish that is often prepared in Italy and Spain. The fish is baked in a crust of salt and egg white to retain its moisture. The fish can be seasoned with various spices and herbs. Sardines Sardines are one of the most popular types of fish in the Mediterranean and are often served grilled or fried. They are marinated in olive oil and lemon juice and seasoned with garlic and parsley. They can be served as a starter or main course.

Mediterranean meat dishes

Mediterranean meat dishes are known for their fresh ingredients and delicious flavors. Here are some of the most popular dishes from this region. One of the most famous Mediterranean meat dishes is Greek moussaka. It consists of layers of eggplants, potatoes, minced meat and tomatoes covered with a creamy béchamel sauce and baked in the oven. The combination of meat and vegetables makes this dish a healthy and hearty meal. Another Greek dish made with meat is souvlaki. It consists of marinated meat skewers that are roasted on a grill or in a pan. The marinade consists of olive oil, lemon juice, garlic and spices and gives the meat a unique Mediterranean flavor. Italian cuisine also has some delicious Mediterranean meat dishes to offer. One of these is osso buco, a classic dish from Lombardy. It consists of cooked veal prepared with tomatoes, carrots, celery and onions. The dish is often served with gremolata, a mixture of lemon zest, garlic and parsley. Another Italian dish made from meat is Saltimbocca alla Romana. It consists of thinly sliced veal topped with sage and Parma ham and fried in butter and white wine. This dish is easy to prepare and has a delicious, spicy flavor. Spanish cuisine also has some Mediterranean meat dishes, including the famous paella. It is a rice dish that is prepared with a variety of ingredients, including chicken, rabbit, pork and seafood. The dish is often seasoned with saffron, which gives it its characteristic yellow color. Another Spanish dish made from meat is chorizo al vino. It consists of chorizo sausage cooked in red wine and spices and is a delicious starter or accompaniment to other dishes. In Turkey, Adana kebab is a well-known meat dish. It consists of minced meat seasoned with onions, peppers, garlic and spices and grilled on a skewer. The dish is often served with rice and salad and is a delicious and filling meal. Another Turkish dish made from meat is köfte. It consists of minced meatballs seasoned with onions, parsley and spices. The meatballs are often placed on skewers and grilled.

Mediterranean poultry dishes

Mediterranean cuisine is known for its fresh ingredients, strong flavors and healthy and tasty dishes. Poultry dishes are a popular choice in Mediterranean cuisine as they provide a light and protein-rich meal. In this article, we will focus on some delicious Mediterranean poultry dishes that are easy to prepare and a great way to enjoy the flavors and ingredients of Mediterranean cuisine. Chicken souvlaki is a Greek dish that consists of marinated chicken pieces grilled on skewers. The marinade consists of olive oil, lemon juice, garlic, oregano and paprika. The skewers are then grilled until the chicken is tender and juicy. The skewers are often served with a fresh tzatziki sauce and a Greek salad. Lemon chicken with olives and capers This dish is a simple but delicious Mediterranean chicken recipe that is marinated with lemon juice, olive oil, garlic, capers and olives. The chicken is then roasted or baked in the oven until golden brown and tender. The dish is often served with a side of rice or couscous and a side of roasted vegetables. Moroccan chicken tagine Moroccan chicken tagine is a traditional dish from North Africa. It is prepared in a special clay pot known as a tagine. The main ingredients are chicken, onions, garlic, coriander, cinnamon, saffron, tomatoes and apricots. The chicken is slowly braised until tender and the dish is often served with couscous and a salad. Lemon rosemary chicken This dish is a classic Mediterranean chicken recipe that is marinated with lemon juice, olive oil, rosemary and garlic. The chicken is then roasted or baked in the oven until golden brown and tender. The dish is often served with a side dish of rice or potatoes and a salad. Turkish chicken kebabs Turkish chicken kebabs are a traditional dish from Turkey consisting of marinated pieces of chicken grilled on skewers. The marinade consists of olive oil, yogurt, garlic, paprika, cumin and coriander. The skewers are then grilled until the chicken is tender and juicy. The skewers are often served with a side dish of rice.

Mediterranean vegetable dishes

Mediterranean cuisine is known for its light and healthy dishes, often made with fresh vegetables and olive oil. In this article, we will look at some of the best Mediterranean vegetable dishes that are easy to prepare and very tasty. Ratatouille Ratatouille is a classic dish from Provence made from tomatoes, eggplants, zucchinis, peppers, onions and garlic. It is often served as a side dish with meat or fish, but it is also delicious as a vegetarian main course. The vegetables are fried in olive oil and then cooked with tomato sauce and spices such as thyme, rosemary and oregano. Caponata Caponata is a Sicilian dish consisting of eggplants, tomatoes, capers, olives and celery. It is often served as a side dish or starter and is very easy to prepare. The eggplants are fried in olive oil and then cooked with the other ingredients and a vinegar and sugar syrup. Vegetable tian tian is a Provençal dish consisting of layers of tomatoes, zucchinis, eggplants and onions. It is often served as a side dish or as a vegetarian main course and is very easy to prepare. The layers of vegetables are seasoned with olive oil and spices such as thyme and rosemary and then baked in the oven. Roasted peppers Roasted peppers are a simple dish consisting of peppers, olive oil, garlic and spices. The peppers are fried in olive oil and then seasoned with garlic and spices such as thyme and oregano. It is a delicious accompaniment to grilled meat or fish. Vegetable spaghetti Vegetable spaghetti is a light and healthy dish consisting of zucchinis, carrots and turnips cut into thin spaghetti strings. The vegetable spaghetti is fried in olive oil and then served with a tomato sauce and spices such as garlic, basil and oregano. Eggplant parmesan Aubergine parmesan is a classic dish from Italian cuisine consisting of fried eggplant slices, tomato sauce, mozzarella and parmesan. The eggplant slices are fried in olive oil and then layered with tomato sauce, mozzarella and Parmesan and baked in the oven. Tomato and cheese gratin Tomato and cheese gratin is a delicious dish consisting of tomatoes, mozzarella and Parmesan. The tomatoes are sliced and then layered with mozzarella and Parmesan in a baking dish and baked in the oven. It is a delicious side dish for grilled meat. Mediterranean legume dishes Mediterranean cuisine is known for its healthy and nutritious legume dishes. Legumes such as beans, lentils, chickpeas and peas are rich in fiber, protein, minerals and vitamins. In this article, I will write 700 words about some of the most popular

Mediterranean legume dishes.

Hummus is a traditional Middle Eastern dish made from pureed chickpeas, tahini (sesame paste), lemon juice, garlic and olive oil. It is a great addition to raw vegetables, sandwiches and as a dip for bread. Falafel Falafel are fried balls of mashed chickpeas or beans, often served in pita bread. They are a popular street food option and are often served with lettuce, tomatoes, cucumber and a sauce made from tahini and lemon juice. Fasolada is a Greek dish made from white beans, tomatoes, carrots, celery, onions and garlic. It is often seasoned with olive oil and herbs and is a hearty dish served especially in winter. Pasta e fagioli is an Italian dish made from pasta and beans. It is often cooked with tomatoes, carrots, celery, onions and garlic and is a simple and delicious dish served in many Italian households. Chana masala is an Indian dish made from chickpeas in a spicy tomato and onion sauce. It is often served with naan bread or rice and is a popular vegetarian dish in India. Lentil soup Lentil soup is a simple dish that is served in many Mediterranean countries. It consists of lentils, tomatoes, carrots, celery, onions and garlic and is often seasoned with olive oil and herbs. Foul medames is an Egyptian dish made from boiled and mashed beans seasoned with garlic, lemon and olive oil. It is often served for breakfast or lunch and eaten with flatbread or pita bread. Cassoulet is a French dish made from white beans, meat (usually sausage or bacon) and vegetables. It is often served in winter and is a hearty dish served with bread or potatoes. Dolmades are stuffed vine leaves that are often found in Mediterranean cuisine. They are filled with a mixture of rice, onions and herbs.

Mediterranean pizza and tarte flambée

Pizza and tarte flambée are two of the most popular dishes in Europe and are often served as a quick and convenient meal on the go or as part of an evening meal. Mediterranean cuisine also has a big influence on these two dishes, as many of the ingredients and flavors come from the coastal regions of the Mediterranean. In this article, we will take a closer look at Mediterranean pizza and tarte flambée and examine what makes them such popular dishes. Mediterranean cuisine is known for its use of fresh and natural ingredients such as olive oil, tomatoes, garlic, onions and herbs such as basil, oregano and rosemary. These ingredients give Mediterranean cuisine a variety of flavors that are both hearty and fresh and are perfect for dishes such as pizza and tarte flambée. Mediterranean pizza is often prepared with a thin crust that is crispy and light. Toppings can vary according to taste, but tomatoes, mozzarella, olives, artichoke hearts and basil are often used. Some variations also contain ham, peppers and onions. Mediterranean pizza can be baked in either a wood-fired or electric oven, but the goal is always the same - to create a crispy, flavorful and satisfying meal. Another popular version of Mediterranean pizza is the so-called "pizza bianca" or "white pizza". This variant is prepared without tomato sauce and is instead spread with garlic oil. Toppings can still be used, but ricotta cheese and parmesan are often added. White pizza is a delicious alternative to traditional pizza and has a creamy and spicy flavor combination. The tarte flambée is a traditional Alsatian dish that has become a popular dish throughout Europe in recent years. Unlike pizza, tarte flambée is made with a thin dough that is traditionally topped with sour cream, onions and bacon. The Mediterranean version of tarte flambée usually contains tomatoes, olive oil, garlic and goat's cheese, and is often garnished with fresh rocket or basil. Tarte flambée is also baked in a wood-fired or electric oven and is a delicious and crispy alternative to pizza. In many Mediterranean countries, tarte flambée is also known as "tarte flambée" and there are many different variations of this dish. Some even include sweet ingredients such as apples or pears sprinkled with cinnamon, which makes for a delicious dessert. One of the best things about Mediterranean pizza and tarte flambée is its versatility.

Burgers and sandwiches

Mediterranean burgers and sandwiches are a delicious alternative to traditional burgers and sandwiches. They are rich in flavor and nutritional benefits that come from the delicious ingredients and healthy way they are prepared. In this article, we'll take a look at what makes Mediterranean cuisine so special, what ingredients are typical and how to use them in burger and sandwich recipes. Mediterranean cuisine has its roots in the countries around the Mediterranean, including Italy, Greece, Spain, France, Morocco and Turkey. The cuisine is known for its abundance of fresh ingredients, such as olive oil, garlic, tomatoes, eggplants and zucchinis, as well as its use of fresh herbs such as basil, oregano and rosemary. It is also known for its use of healthy fats such as olive oil and nuts, as well as its high use of fish and seafood. One of the best ways to enjoy all these delicious Mediterranean ingredients is in a burger or sandwich. Here are some ideas and recipes for Mediterranean burgers and sandwiches for you to try: Falafel Burger Falafel are small, crispy balls of pureed chickpeas that are commonly used in Lebanese and Israeli cuisine. For a Mediterranean falafel burger, you can prepare falafel balls and serve them on a burger bun with fresh tomato slices, cucumber slices, onions, lettuce leaves and a generous helping of tahini sauce. Grilled eggplant burger Aubergines are a staple of Mediterranean cuisine and make a delicious topping for a burger. Slice the eggplants and grill them on both sides until they are soft and tender. Then place a slice of mozzarella cheese on top of the eggplants and allow it to melt. Serve the eggplant slices on a burger bun with fresh basil, tomatoes and a drizzle of balsamic glaze. Tomato and mozzarella sandwich This classic Mediterranean sandwich is simple but incredibly tasty. Slice fresh tomatoes and mozzarella cheese and place them on a slice of freshly baked bread. Then add fresh basil leaves and drizzle with olive oil and balsamic vinegar. Finish off the sandwich with another slice of bread and enjoy! Tuna sandwich Tuna is another popular element of Mediterranean cuisine and makes a delicious sandwich. Mix canned tuna with olive oil, lemon, onions, tomatoes and herbs such as parsley and dill.

Mediterranean sauces and dips

Mediterranean sauces and dips are an important addition to many Mediterranean dishes. They are not only delicious, but also healthy and versatile. Mediterranean cuisine is known for its use of fresh herbs and spices, as well as the healthy fatty acids found in olive oil and nuts. This article introduces some of the most popular Mediterranean sauces and dips. Tzatziki is a Greek sauce made from yogurt, cucumber, garlic and fresh herbs such as dill or mint. It is a cool and refreshing sauce that is often served as a dip for vegetables or as a side dish with grilled meat. Tzatziki is also a healthy choice as it is low in fat and a good source of protein and calcium. Hummus is an oriental sauce made from chickpeas, tahini, olive oil, lemon juice and garlic. It is a creamy and spicy dip that is often served as a snack or appetizer. Hummus is an excellent source of fiber and vegetable protein and contains healthy fats from the olive oil. Pesto Pesto is an Italian sauce made from basil, pine nuts, garlic, olive oil and Parmesan cheese. It is a nutty and aromatic sauce that is often served as a side dish with pasta or as a dip for bread or vegetables. Pesto is a good source of vitamin K, which is important for bone health, as well as healthy fats and protein. Baba Ghanoush is an oriental sauce made from grilled eggplant, tahini, lemon juice, garlic and olive oil. It is a creamy and smoky dip that is often served as an appetizer or side dish with grilled meat. Baba Ghanoush is a good source of fiber, calcium and healthy fats from the olive oil. Romesco is a Spanish sauce made from roasted tomatoes, roasted peppers, almonds, garlic and olive oil. It is a nutty and spicy sauce that is often served as a side dish with grilled vegetables or fish. Romesco is a good source of vitamin C, which is important for the immune system, as well as healthy fats and protein. Aioli is a French sauce made from garlic, egg yolk, olive oil and lemon juice. It is a creamy and flavorful sauce that is often served as a dip for French fries or as an accompaniment to seafood. Aioli is a good source of healthy.

Mediterranean desserts

Mediterranean desserts are famous for their fresh ingredients, light sweetness and delicious combination of flavors and textures. Often made with ingredients such as olive oil, nuts, fruit and honey, these desserts offer a rich variety of delicious options to suit all tastes. Here are some of the best Mediterranean desserts to try: Baklava is a sweet dessert made from puff pastry, often filled with honey and nuts such as pistachios or walnuts. It is a popular choice in the Middle East and Mediterranean and is usually served in small, triangular pieces. Tiramisu is an Italian dessert consisting of layers of ladyfingers and a cream of mascarpone cheese, eggs and sugar. It is usually drizzled with espresso or coffee and dusted with cocoa powder. Crème brûlée is a French dessert consisting of a creamy vanilla custard covered with a crunchy layer of caramelized sugar. It is usually served in small, round bowls and garnished with fresh berries or a sprinkling of cinnamon. Tarte Tatin is a French apple tart in which the pastry is laid over the apples and then baked. After baking, the tart is turned upside down to reveal the apples on top. The tart is usually served warm and can be garnished with a scoop of vanilla ice cream or whipped cream. Churros are a Spanish dessert consisting of deep-fried dough rolled into a tube and sprinkled with sugar. It is usually served with chocolate sauce or dulce de leche. Galaktoboureko is a Greek dessert consisting of a vanilla cream filling in filo pastry and garnished with syrup and cinnamon. It is a delicious choice for anyone who wants a light but sweet dessert. Cannoli are an Italian dessert consisting of a crispy pastry tube filled with a cream of ricotta cheese and sugar. It is usually sprinkled with pistachios or chocolate chips. Crema Catalana is a Spanish dessert that is similar to crème brûlée, but is flavored with orange or lemon zest and cinnamon. The top of the dessert is caramelized and garnished with fresh berries or mint leaves. A sponge roll is a light but sweet dessert consisting of a thin layer of sponge cake.

Food pyramid

The Mediterranean food pyramid is a nutritional concept based on the eating habits of people in Mediterranean countries. It is considered one of the healthiest diets and has gained popularity in recent years. In this article, we will take a closer look at the Mediterranean food pyramid and explain its benefits. The Mediterranean food pyramid consists of a broad base of plant-based foods such as fruit, vegetables, beans, nuts and seeds. This food group forms the largest part of the food pyramid and should therefore make up the largest part of our diet. Plant-based foods are rich in nutrients, fiber, vitamins and minerals and are therefore the basis for a healthy diet. Next in the Mediterranean food pyramid is the group of wholegrain products and pulses. These include wholemeal bread, wholemeal pasta, brown rice and lentils. Wholegrain products are rich in fiber and provide a long-lasting feeling of satiety. Legumes, on the other hand, provide protein and other important nutrients. The next level of the food pyramid is the group of fats. These are healthy fats such as olive oil, nuts and seeds, which are rich in omega-3 fatty acids and therefore support heart health. However, portions should also be kept in mind here, as healthy fats also have a high energy density. Next comes the group of dairy products and eggs. These include yogurt, cheese and eggs. Dairy products and eggs are rich in protein and important nutrients such as calcium. However, you should also keep an eye on your portions here, as dairy products and eggs also contain saturated fatty acids. The group of meat products and sweets forms the top of the food pyramid. This includes meat, sausages, chocolate, sweets and soft drinks. These foods should only be consumed in moderation as they are high in saturated fat, sugar and calories. The Mediterranean diet pyramid is based on the eating habits of people in Mediterranean countries and is therefore rich in healthy nutrients while reducing the consumption of unhealthy foods. There are numerous studies that prove the benefits of the Mediterranean diet. Among other things, it is said to reduce the risk of heart disease, diabetes, cancer and Alzheimer's disease.

The Mediterranean lifestyle

Exercise and relaxation The Mediterranean lifestyle is a healthy and sustainable lifestyle that focuses on diet, exercise and relaxation. It is a lifestyle that is mainly practiced in countries around the Mediterranean Sea, including Spain, France, Italy, Greece and Turkey. The Mediterranean lifestyle has been declared an intangible cultural heritage by UNESCO and has become popular worldwide due to its health benefits. In this article, we focus on exercise and relaxation, the two essential pillars of the Mediterranean lifestyle. Exercise: Exercise is an important part of the Mediterranean lifestyle. Unlike intense workouts at the gym, exercise in the Mediterranean lifestyle is about moving regularly and staying physically active. People in Mediterranean countries tend to walk, cycle or swim a lot, rather than focusing on fast and strenuous exercise. This type of exercise is also suitable for people with limited physical mobility. Another form of exercise in the Mediterranean lifestyle is dance. It is a fun and creative way to stay physically active. Dance is also an important part of the culture in Mediterranean countries, and many people enjoy dancing in groups or at festivals. One important thing to understand about exercise in the Mediterranean lifestyle is that there is no strict routine. People in these countries incorporate exercise into their daily lives by, for example, walking to work, climbing stairs or gardening. The goal is to keep the body moving and stay active rather than focusing on strenuous workouts. Relaxation: Relaxation is just as important as exercise in the Mediterranean lifestyle. People in these countries have a balanced work-life balance, which allows them to de-stress and relax. One of the best ways to relax is meditation. It is a simple and effective way to calm the mind and relax. People in Mediterranean countries often practice meditation in the form of prayers or spiritual practices. Another way to relax is to read. Reading can transport us to other worlds and help us to relax our minds. People in Mediterranean countries often have a culture of reading, where they regularly take time to read books. Another form of relaxation in the Mediterranean lifestyle is socializing. People in these countries enjoy spending time with friends and family and socializing. It is a way to relax the mind and make social connections.

Diet during pregnancy and breastfeeding

The Mediterranean diet, traditionally practiced in countries such as Italy, Greece and Spain, is known for its health benefits. A growing number of studies show that the Mediterranean diet can also be beneficial during pregnancy and breastfeeding. In this article, we will look at the benefits of the Mediterranean diet for pregnant and breastfeeding women and provide some recommendations on how to incorporate this diet into your daily routine. What is the Mediterranean diet? The Mediterranean diet is based on a diet rich in fruit, vegetables, whole grains, nuts, seeds and healthy fats such as olive oil and fish. This diet is low in red meat, processed foods and sugar. It is also recommended to drink wine in moderation and to watch your intake of dairy products. This diet has been shown to be beneficial for cardiovascular health, weight management and overall quality of life. Benefits of the Mediterranean diet during pregnancy During pregnancy, women have an increased need for nutrients to support the growth and development of the fetus. The Mediterranean diet provides an abundance of nutrients, including omega-3 fatty acids, folate, iron, calcium and vitamin D, which are crucial for a healthy pregnancy and fetal development. A study published in the American Journal of Clinical Nutrition found that women who practiced a Mediterranean diet during pregnancy had a lower risk of pregnancy complications such as gestational diabetes and pre-eclampsia. The Mediterranean diet was also associated with a lower risk of premature birth. Benefits of the Mediterranean diet during breastfeeding. During breastfeeding, it is important that women eat a balanced diet to maximize the quality and quantity of breast milk. The Mediterranean diet can help meet the nutritional needs of the breastfeeding mother while promoting the health of the baby. A study published in the Journal of Human Lactation found that breastfeeding women who practiced a Mediterranean diet had higher concentrations of omega-3 fatty acids in their breast milk, which are important for the baby's brain development. Another study published in the International Breastfeeding Journal found that women who practiced a Mediterranean diet had higher milk production than women who practiced a Western diet. Recommendations for implementing the Mediterranean diet during pregnancy and breastfeeding.

Diet for children and adolescents

The Mediterranean diet is a diet that is mainly practiced in countries around the Mediterranean. This diet is rich in fruits, vegetables, whole grains, nuts, legumes and olive oil, while the consumption of red meat, sugar and processed foods is limited. In recent years, the Mediterranean diet has been shown to offer numerous health benefits, including reducing the risk of heart disease, cancer and diabetes. But what about the effects of the Mediterranean diet on children and adolescents? Children and adolescents have special nutritional needs as they are in a phase of growth and physical development. A balanced diet is therefore particularly important to ensure that they get all the nutrients they need. The Mediterranean diet can be a good option here. Studies have shown that children who follow a Mediterranean diet have a lower risk of obesity and overweight compared to children who eat a different diet. The Mediterranean diet also appears to have a positive effect on cholesterol levels. Fruit and vegetables are an important part of the Mediterranean diet. These should be included in every meal. Children and teenagers should be encouraged to eat a variety of fruit and vegetables to ensure they get all the vitamins and minerals they need. It is important that fruit and vegetables are served in an appealing and tasty way to keep young people interested. For example, fruit and vegetables can be offered in the form of smoothies or salads. Whole grain products are another important part of the Mediterranean diet. These are an important source of fiber, which helps to keep the intestines healthy. Children and teenagers should be encouraged to eat whole grain products instead of refined carbohydrates such as white bread, pasta and rice. One way to do this is to serve whole grain bread instead of white bread and use whole grain pasta instead of regular pasta. Another important feature of the Mediterranean diet is legumes such as beans, lentils and chickpeas. These are an excellent source of vegetable protein and fiber. Pulses can be prepared in a variety of ways, for example as a soup, stew or salad. Olive oil is another important feature of the Mediterranean diet. It contains healthy fats that are important for the growth and development of children and adolescents. Olive oil can be used to flavor salads or as a substitute for butter or margarine.

The Mediterranean diet for diabetes

Diabetes is a chronic disease characterized by high blood sugar levels that can lead to serious complications such as cardiovascular disease, kidney disease, blindness and amputations. A healthy diet is an important part of diabetes management and can help control blood glucose levels and prevent complications. A diet based on the Mediterranean diet can be particularly beneficial. The Mediterranean diet is a way of eating traditionally practiced in countries around the Mediterranean such as Italy, Greece and Spain. It is rich in vegetables, fruit, whole grains, olive oil, fish and lean meat. The diet is also characterized by moderate amounts of wine and cheese. The Mediterranean diet has been shown to be effective in preventing cardiovascular disease, cancer and other chronic diseases. There is also evidence that it can be helpful in controlling diabetes. A study published in the New England Journal of Medicine found that the Mediterranean diet can reduce the risk of type 2 diabetes by more than 50 percent. Another study published in the Journal of the American College of Cardiology showed that the Mediterranean diet led to a significant improvement in blood sugar levels, blood pressure and cholesterol levels in patients with type 2 diabetes. The Mediterranean diet is rich in fibre, which can help stabilize blood sugar levels. Fiber slows the digestion and absorption of carbohydrates, which can help slow the rise in blood sugar levels after a meal. Fiber can also help lower cholesterol and reduce the risk of cardiovascular disease in people with diabetes. The Mediterranean diet is based on the use of healthy oils such as olive oil. Olive oil is a source of monounsaturated fatty acids, which can help control blood sugar levels. Monounsaturated fatty acids are also known to lower the risk of cardiovascular disease and stroke. A study published in the American Journal of Clinical Nutrition found that a diet rich in olive oil can lead to a significant improvement in blood sugar levels and cholesterol levels in people with diabetes. The Mediterranean diet is also rich in omega-3 fatty acids, which are mainly found in fish such as salmon, tuna and sardines. Omega-3 fatty acids can help to reduce inflammation.

The Mediterranean diet for cardiovascular disease

The Mediterranean diet is a diet characterized by a rich variety of fruits, vegetables, whole grains, legumes, fish, olive oil and nuts. This diet is often considered one of the healthiest diets and has been shown in numerous studies to reduce the risk of heart disease and stroke. Cardiovascular disease is one of the leading causes of death worldwide. These diseases are often caused by a combination of risk factors such as high blood pressure, high cholesterol, obesity and diabetes. A healthy diet can help to reduce the risk of cardiovascular disease. The Mediterranean diet is rich in fiber, vitamins, minerals and antioxidants. The diet is low in saturated fats and trans fats, which are found in many processed foods and can contribute to elevated cholesterol levels. Instead, the Mediterranean diet is based on the consumption of unsaturated fatty acids from olive oil and nuts, which can help to lower cholesterol levels. A 2013 study found that a Mediterranean diet can reduce the risk of heart attacks, strokes and deaths from heart disease by around 30 percent. Another study from 2018 showed that a Mediterranean diet can reduce the risk of cardiovascular disease in people at high risk by around 25 percent. A Mediterranean diet also has positive effects on blood pressure. High blood pressure is an important risk factor for heart disease and strokes. A 2016 study showed that a Mediterranean diet can lower systolic blood pressure (the upper value) by an average of 3.5 mmHg. A Mediterranean diet can also help to control weight. Obesity is another risk factor for cardiovascular disease. A study from 2010 showed that a Mediterranean diet can help to reduce body weight and reduce waist circumference. In addition to diet, physical activity and a healthy lifestyle are also important factors in the prevention of cardiovascular disease. However, a Mediterranean diet can help to improve health and reduce the risk of heart disease and stroke. A Mediterranean diet can also be beneficial for people with existing cardiovascular disease.

Diet for cancer

The Mediterranean diet is a way of eating characterized by the consumption of fresh fruits and vegetables, olive oil, nuts, fish and whole grains. This type of diet has long been associated with a number of health benefits, including a lower risk of heart disease, diabetes and stroke. In recent years, the Mediterranean diet has also been shown to have a positive impact on cancer. Cancer is a complex disease characterized by the uncontrolled growth and spread of abnormal cells in the body. There are different types of cancer, but some common features such as inflammation and oxidative stress can contribute to the onset and development of cancer. A healthy diet can help minimize these risk factors and thus reduce the risk of cancer. A number of studies have shown that the Mediterranean diet has a protective effect against cancer. For example, a 2018 study found that people who followed the Mediterranean diet had a lower risk of developing various cancers such as breast cancer, colorectal cancer and prostate cancer. Another report from 2015 found that the Mediterranean diet was also associated with a better survival rate in people with cancer. One of the main components of the Mediterranean diet is olive oil. Olive oil contains healthy fats, including monounsaturated fatty acids, which are known for lowering cholesterol levels and reducing the risk of inflammation in the body. In addition, olive oil also contains antioxidants such as polyphenols, which can reduce inflammation and oxidative stress in the body, which can be responsible for the development of cancer. Another important component of the Mediterranean diet is the consumption of fish, especially oily fish species such as salmon and tuna. Fish is an excellent source of omega-3 fatty acids, which are known to reduce inflammation and oxidative stress in the body. There is also some evidence that omega-3 fatty acids can help inhibit the growth and spread of cancer cells. In addition to olive oil and fish, the

Mediterranean diet also recommends eating plenty of fruit and vegetables. These foods are rich in antioxidants, vitamins and minerals, all of which can help reduce inflammation in the body and lower the risk of cancer. For example, a 2020 study found that eating fruit and vegetables was associated with a lower risk of cancer.

Diet for Alzheimer's disease

The Mediterranean diet is a diet rich in fruits, vegetables, whole grains, nuts, legumes, fish and olive oil. This diet has attracted a lot of attention in recent years as it offers numerous health benefits, particularly for the cardiovascular system. There is also evidence that the Mediterranean diet can help reduce the risk of developing Alzheimer's disease. Alzheimer's is a progressive neurodegenerative disease that causes the loss of nerve cells in the brain. Symptoms include memory loss, confusion, difficulty performing everyday tasks and speech difficulties. The disease currently has no cure and there are limited treatment options. Therefore, it is crucial to take preventative measures to reduce the risk of developing Alzheimer's. A 2017 study investigated the effects of the Mediterranean diet on brain function in older people. The results showed that a Mediterranean diet was associated with a lower risk of cognitive impairment and a lower rate of brain decline. Another study from 2018 examined the effects of a Mediterranean diet on brain volume in older adults. The results showed that participants who followed a Mediterranean diet had greater brain volume compared to those who did not. There are several reasons why the Mediterranean diet may help prevent Alzheimer's disease. First, the Mediterranean diet is rich in antioxidants, which can help reduce free radical damage. Free radicals are molecules that can damage cells in the body and can contribute to the development of Alzheimer's disease. Secondly, the Mediterranean diet is rich in omega-3 fatty acids, which are important for brain health. Omega-3 fatty acids contribute to the formation of cell membranes in the brain and can also reduce inflammation in the body. Inflammation is a possible cause of the development of Alzheimer's disease. Thirdly, the Mediterranean diet is rich in carbohydrates with a low glycemic index. Low glycemic index foods are converted into glucose more slowly and lead to a slower release of insulin. A high concentration of insulin in the body can cause inflammation and oxidative damage in the brain and contribute to the development of Alzheimer's disease. The Mediterranean diet for overweight and obesity The Mediterranean diet is a way of eating that was first observed in Mediterranean countries in the 1960s. Since then, it has attracted a lot of attention due to its numerous health benefits, especially in relation to overweight and obesity. The Mediterranean diet is rich in fruits, vegetables, whole grains, olive oil, nuts, fish and lean meats. It is often considered one of the healthiest diets and can help reduce the risk of cardiovascular disease, diabetes and cancer. In this article, we will take a closer look at the Mediterranean diet and its use for overweight and obesity.

The Mediterranean diet and its benefits for overweight and obesity

A Mediterranean diet has been shown to be effective in the prevention and treatment of obesity and overweight. A 2018 study published in the Journal of Nutrition showed that the Mediterranean diet led to significant weight loss in overweight women. Another 2016 study published in the American Journal of Clinical Nutrition found that a Mediterranean diet caused weight loss and improved cardiovascular risk factors in obese men and women. The Mediterranean diet can also help rid the body of inflammation associated with obesity and overweight. A 2010 study published in the Journal of the American Medical Association showed that the Mediterranean diet led to a significant decrease in inflammatory markers in overweight and obese individuals. There is also evidence that a Mediterranean diet can reduce the risk of diabetes. A 2014 study published in the New England Journal of Medicine found that a Mediterranean diet significantly reduced the risk of developing type 2 diabetes in people at high risk of cardiovascular disease. The Mediterranean diet and its main characteristics The Mediterranean diet is characterized by the consumption of fruits, vegetables, whole grains, olive oil, nuts, fish and lean meat. The diet is also based on the consumption of fresh fruit and vegetables and the use of olive oil as the main source of fat. A Mediterranean diet also includes a moderate amount of wine. Research has shown that moderate consumption of wine (especially red wine) can be associated with a lower incidence of cardiovascular disease and lower mortality.

Diet for arthritis and joint disease

The Mediterranean diet is a way of eating based on the culinary habits of people in the Mediterranean region. It is rich in vegetables, fruit, fish, whole grains and unsaturated fatty acids from olive oil and nuts. Numerous studies have shown that the Mediterranean diet is associated with a number of health benefits, including a reduction in the risk of cardiovascular disease, diabetes and certain types of cancer. Another interesting application of the Mediterranean diet is its potential role in the treatment of arthritis and joint disease. Arthritis is an inflammatory disease that affects joints and cartilage, causing pain and stiffness. In many cases, a change in dietary habits can help to reduce inflammation and associated pain. A Mediterranean diet can help, as it is rich in anti-inflammatory nutrients such as omega-3 fatty acids and antioxidants. A 2017 study published in the American Journal of Clinical Nutrition investigated the link between the Mediterranean diet and joint disease in women. The results showed that women who adhered to a Mediterranean diet had a lower risk of developing rheumatoid arthritis than women who did not follow this diet. The researchers suggested that the anti-inflammatory properties of the Mediterranean diet may help to reduce the development of joint disease. Another study from 2018, published in the journal Nutrients, investigated the link between the Mediterranean diet and the treatment of osteoarthritis. The researchers found that the Mediterranean diet can help reduce the pain and inflammation associated with osteoarthritis. The results suggest that the Mediterranean diet can be used as an adjunct to conventional osteoarthritis treatment. There are several reasons why the Mediterranean diet may be helpful for arthritis and joint disease. For one, it is rich in omega-3 fatty acids, which have anti-inflammatory properties. Fish such as salmon, mackerel and sardines are good sources of omega-3 fatty acids. Secondly, the Mediterranean diet contains many antioxidants that can help reduce inflammation in the body. Fruit and vegetables, especially berries and green leafy vegetables, are rich in antioxidants. Nuts and olive oil are also important components of the Mediterranean diet and contain many healthy fats.

Diet for skin diseases

The Mediterranean diet is a diet based on the traditional eating habits of people in the countries around the Mediterranean. This diet is known for its health benefits, particularly in relation to the prevention of cardiovascular disease, diabetes and cancer. However, the Mediterranean diet has also been shown to be beneficial in the prevention and treatment of skin conditions. Skin diseases are a common problem that affects people of all ages. Most skin conditions are not life-threatening, but they can have a major impact on life and affect quality of life. A healthy diet can help reduce the risk of skin conditions and promote healing. The Mediterranean diet is a diet rich in fruits, vegetables, whole grains, nuts and seeds, healthy fats and lean proteins. These foods are rich in important nutrients such as antioxidants, vitamins and minerals that can help boost the immune system and reduce inflammation. Inflammatory skin conditions such as psoriasis and eczema can be caused by an inflammatory response in the body. An anti-inflammatory diet such as the Mediterranean diet can help to reduce inflammation in the body, which can have a positive effect on the skin. A 2018 study published in the Journal of the American Academy of Dermatology found that the Mediterranean diet can be effective in the treatment of psoriasis. The study found that patients who followed the Mediterranean diet showed a significant improvement in their symptoms. Another benefit of the Mediterranean diet for skin conditions is its ability to regulate blood sugar levels. High blood sugar levels can lead to inflammation in the body, which can exacerbate skin conditions such as acne and rosacea. The Mediterranean diet is high in complex carbohydrates from whole grains, which can slowly raise blood sugar levels and thus reduce inflammation. A 2019 study published in the Journal of the Academy of Nutrition and Dietetics found that the Mediterranean diet can be effective in preventing and treating acne. The Mediterranean diet is also rich in healthy fats such as olive oil and fish oil, which contain omega-3 fatty acids. Omega-3 fatty acids have anti-inflammatory properties and can help to balance hormones in the body, which can be beneficial for skin conditions such as acne and rosacea.

The Mediterranean diet for sleep disorders

The Mediterranean diet is a way of eating that is widespread in the countries around the Mediterranean. It is characterized by the consumption of lots of vegetables, fruit, whole grains, nuts, fish and olive oil and is considered one of the healthiest diets in the world. A variety of studies have shown that the Mediterranean diet has many health benefits, including improved heart health, reduced inflammation and a lower likelihood of developing diabetes or cancer. In addition, the Mediterranean diet can also help to alleviate sleep disorders. Insomnia is a common problem that affects millions of people worldwide. There are many reasons why people may have sleep problems, including stress, anxiety, depression, physical ailments and a poor diet. A poor diet can increase the risk of sleep disorders, as certain nutrients and foods can affect the brain and body and interfere with sleep. The Mediterranean diet is rich in certain nutrients that have been linked to better sleep quality. For example, the Mediterranean diet contains many vitamins and minerals, such as magnesium, calcium and vitamin B6, which can help regulate sleep. Magnesium, found in nuts, whole grains and leafy greens, can help relax the body and promote muscle relaxation, which in turn can lead to better sleep. Calcium, found in dairy products, green vegetables and sardines, can also help regulate sleep by promoting the release of melatonin, a hormone responsible for the sleep-wake cycle. Another important component of the Mediterranean diet that can help improve sleep is omega-3 fatty acids. Omega-3 fatty acids are found in fish, especially fatty fish such as salmon and sardines. They can help reduce inflammation in the body and reduce stress, which can contribute to improved sleep. A 2014 study found that increasing omega-3 consumption in older adults led to a significant improvement in sleep quality. A Mediterranean diet can also help regulate blood sugar levels, which in turn can contribute to better sleep. A high intake of refined carbohydrates and sugar can lead to an increase in blood sugar levels, which can lead to a disturbed sleep-wake cycle.

Conclusion: The Mediterranean diet as a long-term dietary change

The Mediterranean diet has received a lot of attention in recent years as a healthy and sustainable dietary change. It is based on the traditional eating habits of Mediterranean countries, which are rich in vegetables, fruit, nuts, pulses, fish and olive oil. There are a variety of scientific studies that have shown that a Mediterranean diet is associated with numerous health benefits, including a reduction in the risk of heart disease, stroke, diabetes and cancer. A Mediterranean diet can be beneficial in the long term as it is based on a healthy and balanced diet that contains a variety of nutrients. Unlike many other diets, the Mediterranean diet does not emphasize a radical restriction of foods, but focuses on a sustainable change in eating habits. This means that a Mediterranean diet is easier to maintain in the long term than other diets that are designed for short-term results. A Mediterranean diet can also have a positive effect on weight. Because the Mediterranean diet is based on healthy fats, whole grains and protein-rich foods, it can help increase satiety and reduce cravings. Combined with regular physical activity, a Mediterranean diet can help you achieve and maintain a healthy weight. Another strength of the Mediterranean diet is its flexibility and adaptability to individual needs and preferences. There are no strict rules or prohibitions, which means that people can adapt the Mediterranean diet to their cultural preferences and circumstances. For example, a vegetarian or vegan approach can be incorporated into a Mediterranean dietary pattern by incorporating plant-based protein sources such as legumes, nuts and seeds. Although the Mediterranean diet offers many benefits, there are also some challenges to implementing it. A Mediterranean diet requires time and preparation to prepare and cook fresh foods. Buying fresh ingredients can also be more expensive than buying processed foods. In addition, it can be difficult to maintain a Mediterranean dietary change in a society dominated by fast food and processed foods. Another challenge is that the Mediterranean diet may not be suitable for everyone. People with specific dietary needs, such as those with food intolerances, may not be able to follow the Mediterranean diet.

Imprint:

Marie Moreno
Am Anger 3
06869 Coswig
Germany
Luna-Publishing.de